MW00872907

the beautiful scoliotic back
2nd Edition – Revised and Expanded

erin myers

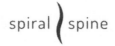
spiral spine

The Beautiful Scoliotic Back

2nd Edition – Revised and Expanded

Copyright © 2014 Erin Myers, Spiral Spine

ISBN-13: 978-1-50007739-0-8

Cover design: 12 South Music
Cover photos: Angela Marie Photography
Interior layout: Lighthouse24
Interior photos: Erin Myers, Spiral Spine

table of contents

a note from Erin

Since I first published *The Beautiful Scoliotic Back* a few years ago, I've received tremendous feedback from people all over the world, from all walks of the scoliotic life. My ever-changing journey has allowed me to hone the focus of *The Beautiful Scoliotic Back* to meet the initial needs of parents and children after they get the hard news of a scoliosis diagnosis. At that tough time, they deeply need to be introduced to a softer side of scoliosis. This is now the focus of *The Beautiful Scoliotic Back*.

My own, ever-changing journey with scoliosis has allowed me to specifically refine the focus of this book to meet the initial needs of parents and children after receiving the hard news of a scoliosis diagnosis. At that tough and confusing time, facts appear cold and options appear to be few. I want to introduce you to a softer, more understanding side of scoliosis. What you really want to hear is that it's going to be OK. I know. I've been there. I am there. I walk alongside my clients every day and assure them that it's going to be OK.

So, grab your favorite cup of tea and let's have a heart-to-heart conversation about scoliosis. I'll tell you what my years of research and experience have led me to believe, and I'll share with you my story, and the stories of my clients – valuable insight that will allow you to come up with your own plan to deal with your scoliosis. It's going to be OK. Really.

introduction

I think the back is the most beautiful part of the human body, even ones that are a bit different because of the spiral spines that are etched into them.

My passion, love and admiration for backs began when I was enrolled in a classical ballet school during high school. For hours each day, I'd be in a room with a bunch of other sweaty teenaged girls wearing tights and a leotard. Our leotards were low in the back so I could see the gorgeous, defined muscles in each girl's back. I actually remember looking at a girl's back one day and thinking that a particular muscle group looked like a beautiful Christmas tree stretching across her back. Who knew that many years later, I'd be instructing anatomy classes and teaching others that the Christmas tree was actually the rhomboid muscles?

People often ask me how I came to specialize in scoliotic corrective exercise. The simple answer is that scoliosis doesn't scare me. I've worked with bodies that, quite frankly, scare a lot of other body practitioners like children, amputees, and individuals who are grossly overweight. Others are frightened because they don't know what to do with these clients, they're afraid of hurting them or they don't want to make their conditions worse. I've taken courses specifically on scoliosis, sifted through mounds of scoliosis research, and experimented firsthand with what works and what doesn't by practicing on my own body and my clients' bodies.

I have a deep passion for teaching others about scoliosis: clients, parents whose children have been diagnosed with scoliosis, Pilates teachers, you name it. Oftentimes, people shy away from talking about scoliosis as if the very word is too forbidden or scary to discuss. I'm here to tell you that's just not so.

I have scoliosis and it hasn't stopped me from living an abundantly full life. I was diagnosed at the age of 14 with a 17 degree "S" curve in my spine. Through different hormonal stages in my life, my scoliosis has worsened. Yet I've danced with the Radio City Rockettes, owned a successful Pilates studio, and birthed two healthy boys. A diagnosis of scoliosis is nothing to be scared of and it certainly isn't the end of the world.

1) learning to own your scoliosis

Rather than try and fill your head with a bunch of medical jargon to describe exactly what happens to a person physically with scoliosis, I want to simply inform you about scoliosis as a whole. Just like I tell all of my scoliotic clients, I want you to learn how to *own* your scoliosis. Some days your back will feel good, and some days, not so much. No matter what, you'll live with this for the rest of your life, so it's best to understand what's going on with your body.

I like to say that scoliosis is 16-dimensional. Scoliosis doesn't just affect the two-dimensional "C" or "S" side shift of the spine, or even just the three-dimensional rotation of the spine, it affects *so* much more. Scoliosis affects the placement of the head, how the arms hang off the ribcage, even the placement of the feet. It can also greatly affect one's emotional and psychological outlook on life.

Here's a simple way to visualize scoliosis: Think of your ribcage as a house. The foundation on which the house (ribcage) was built is crooked, making for a crooked house. From the crooked house, you sometimes get a crooked rooftop line (shoulders), and the windows may be uneven (shoulder-blades). Since the foundation of the house is a bit crooked, the basement (pelvis) may be a bit off-kilter, as well.

For example, my pelvis is rotated in the opposite direction from my ribcage, while some scoliotic people have their pelvises rotating in the same direction. One of my legs is more turned out than the other, as well. All of this is affected by my 'crooked house' and 'crooked foundation' (aka scoliosis).

When I was younger, I used to think that one of my breasts was larger than the other. Once I learned more about my scoliosis, I realized that it was actually my ribcage (my house) that was rotated and that my breasts were not different sizes.

Now, let's take this a step further: here is a picture of my back that was taken almost 10 years ago, a few months after I finished my second season dancing with the Radio City Rockettes. See how different the right and left sides of my body are?

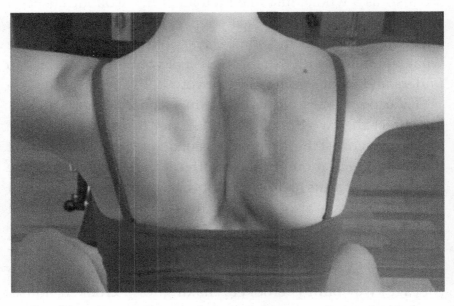

In this picture, I was doing my best to be as straight as possible. It's obvious that my spine is not in the center of my back, as it curves to the right. If the picture went down even further, you'd notice my spine curving a bit to the left at the bottom. Because my spine curves to the right, the muscles directly to the right of the curve look beefier than the muscles on my left side.

You'll also notice that my right shoulder is higher than my left and my neck and shoulder muscles are more developed on the right side. The bottoms of my armpits are uneven. They're even shaped differently. My left side is lower than my right.

Interestingly, my legs are crisscrossed in the picture and even my legs are uneven. My left knee is higher than my right. More of my left leg is shown than my right because my ribcage is shifted to the right, causing part of my right leg to be hidden. All thanks to my spiral spine.

Note that I'm intentionally being really picky with the analysis of my body, as most people don't even notice these differences. When I was dancing with the Rockettes, no one ever said, "Hmmmm, I notice that the third girl from the left has scoliosis." No way! No one ever noticed that something was different about me.

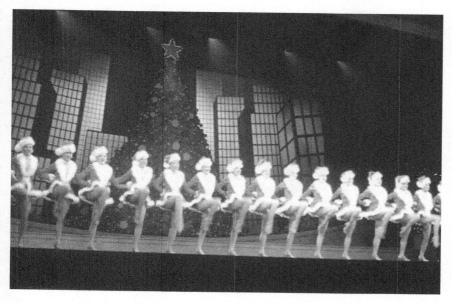

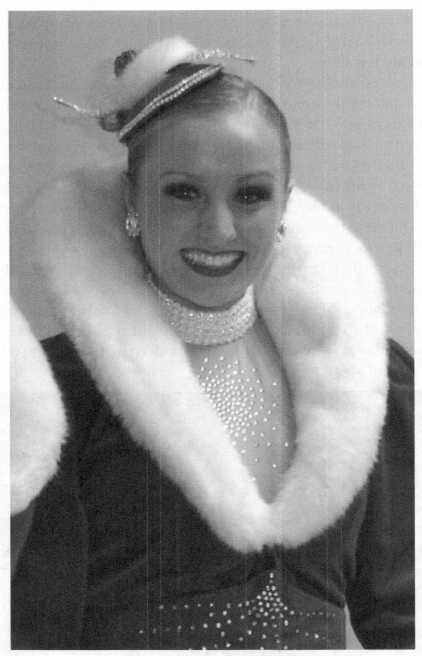

Erin Myers, Radio City Rockette, 2005.

As we continue on this journey and you start to analyze your own body, know that most people will never even realize you have scoliosis either.

Here's another photo of me wearing a t-shirt that was taken a few years after I opened my first Pilates studio, and few months after giving birth to my first child. In spite of all my years of dancing, Pilates, my pregnancy, and giving birth, my body still showed the same scoliotic shifts.

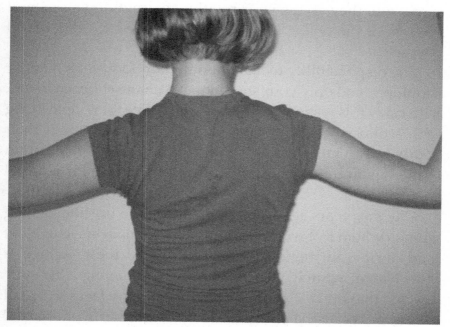

Yep, scoliosis is part of who I am.

So, what does owning your scoliosis mean? Simply put, it means that you not only know the medical degree of your curvature and rotation, but you know what that degree of curvature and rotation feels like in your body. You know how your body as a whole feels on a good day and a not-so-good day.

There will be days, and even periods of your life, where you will feel quite scoliotic and twisted up. But because you've taken steps to *own* your scoliosis, you'll know what your scoliosis feels like on a good day, which will empower you to take action on days when it doesn't feel so good. Later in the book, I'll offer some suggestions as to different types of practitioners who can help you unwind.

Your physician will most likely *not* be the one to tell you how to unwind. In my experience, physicians will take X-rays of your spine to determine the degree of your curve, but rarely will they assess your rotation, or anything else about the rest of the body. This is what you need to learn about yourself.

The responsibility to learn about your body rests on your shoulders, and only your shoulders. Even the children I work with carry this responsibility. It's imperative for people living with scoliosis to understand that no one cares about their bodily health more than they do. Coming to that realization is the beginning of a bright future of living with a spiral spine.

One day years ago, "Naomi,"* one of the precious young women whom I've worked with for years, made me laugh out loud during our regular private lesson. At the mere age of nine, Naomi astutely told me that she was having a 'twisted' day and that the fascia in her ribcage was tight. I was so proud of Naomi because she was learning to own her scoliosis and reach out for help when she deemed it necessary.

While pregnant with my first son, Levi, my spine was almost straight. It was amazing. My longtime massage therapist was stunned at my back during that time. On the other hand, a year after I gave birth to Levi, my back wound up into a tight corkscrew again. Interestingly, my spine never unwound when I was pregnant with my second son, Asher, and has stayed quite bound ever since.

But because I had an acute sense of how my body felt and functioned, I was able to start a new therapy approach to stop the ongoing spiraling of my spine.

I want you to be able to monitor your scoliosis throughout your entire lifetime, even as hormonal and lifestyle changes occur. You must take charge of your body, and recognize when your body doesn't feel right. Only then can you take proactive steps to help it feel and function better.

*All clients' names have been changed in respect of their privacy.

2) emotionally dealing with scoliosis

I have blue eyes. I have size nine feet. I have two legs and two arms. I have scoliosis. It's just part of my body and needs to be treated as such. Scoliosis may need a bit more attention than, say, my size nine feet (which have their own problems...like painful bunions), but nonetheless, it's still just part of my bodily make-up. Most of us have aspects of our bodies that we're sensitive about. For some, it's the shape of their legs and for others, it might be acne that causes embarrassment. We all tend to have body issues, which trigger emotional responses.

For many of my clients, their scoliosis triggers an emotional response. As a practitioner, I work really hard not to use emotional words with my clients, like "weak" and "tight." I instead use words like "short," "long," "beefy," "chord-like" or "gummy" when speaking of different parts of the body and how they look and feel. This way, it doesn't become emotional when assessing a client's scoliotic body in person – especially when it is a young, hormone-raging, pre-pubescent, female client. I've worked with clients who've spiraled down into deep depression because their doctor told them they had scoliosis. It is extremely challenging to deal with clients like this because I can't just work on their bodies – I have to tend to their emotional scoliotic scars, as well.

For example, one day Naomi, the client I spoke of earlier, came in for her regular lesson a little down-in-the-dumps. Naomi's mom stepped out of the Pilates studio to make a phone call, giving Naomi and me a chance to chat. She told me she was the only student at school with a roller backpack (one with wheels on the bottom and a handle that extends so you can roll the backpack on the ground instead of carrying it on your back) and she was embarrassed. To an adult, this would be no big deal, but to a hormone-raging, 13 year-old girl, it was enough to emotionally shut her down.

What Naomi didn't know that was that a few years earlier, when her scoliotic curve was progressing, it was me who had advised her mom to buy her that roller backpack. I firmly stand by that recommendation because at the time, it was needed to relieve her of the uneven strain of trucking a 20 pound-traditional backpack on her back during long hours at school. Now, however, a few years had passed and Naomi's scoliosis was no longer progressing.

Right after this particular lesson, I emailed Naomi's mom. I told her that in my professional opinion, the blue (non-roller) backpack from the most recent Lands' End catalog would solve all of Naomi's scoliotic issues (I was joking, of course). It was the exact backpack Naomi had told me she wanted so she would fit in at school. I told Naomi's mom that scoliosis makes her daughter different enough, and that this one small adjustment would be more beneficial than detrimental. This is an example of the emotional side of scoliosis.

And by the way, this is one of the rare occasions where I've dealt with scoliosis in a lighter manner. As a rule of thumb, it's nothing to joke about. People with scoliosis and parents of children with scoliosis need to be dealt with lovingly and encouragingly. Scoliosis is something they will live and deal with forever and they need continuous, positive, emotional fuel for the long road ahead. They don't need to be the brunt of jokes.

On the other end of the spectrum are those who use the scoliosis card as a lifelong crutch. I was in a Bible study class one day with "Margaret," a woman in her mid-50s who was fairly overweight and shuffled along slowly with a cane. Margaret knew I was a Pilates instructor, but knew nothing beyond that.

One day, before our study class started, I asked Margaret to tell me her health story. She became wide-eyed and dramatic: "I have scoliosis," she whispered. "My doctor said I won't be able to walk one day." I sat there absolutely dumbfounded. For one of the only times in my life, I remained speechless. I don't know exactly what her doctor had told her, but it was enough for her to give up hope and throw in the towel on her scoliosis. Because her mind was set on the final outcome, I didn't even tell her that working with people with scoliosis was my specialty. And for the record, losing the ability to walk is not a side effect or final outcome of scoliosis.

Something that brought Margaret's health story to mind was that she never mentioned scoliotic surgery, which must have meant her scoliosis curve wasn't that severe. If her scoliosis was bad enough that organ function was affected, I'm sure her physician would have recommended surgery. Interestingly, I later found out that Margaret's own husband was a physician. The apparent lack of optimism, which seemed to stem from the physicians in Margaret's life, may have sabotaged any hope she may have had. It saddens me that Margaret gave up hope, especially since pathologically, her scoliosis couldn't have been that severe.

I had another client, "Linda," who made me furious every time she entered my Pilates studio. Whenever Linda walked in, I had to put on my theatre face and beam my Rockette smile as I silently growled at her in my head. Linda was in her late 20s and had a handicapped-parking sticker for her car (prescribed by a physician)...for her scoliosis. To see her parking in the handicapped-parking space right in front of the studio and coming in to take an hour-long Pilates mat class was almost unbearable. Her back wasn't bad enough for surgery but somehow she had played the scoliotic card well enough to get a physician to prescribe a handicapped-sticker for her car so she didn't have to walk as far when running errands because "it was too much work." *Argh!*

She also suffered from depression, which caused her to flunk out of her pre-med classes in college. Linda openly called herself "The Hunchback of Notre Dame," and would always wear a coat in public to hide her scoliosis. Linda blamed scoliosis for the decline in her life and it made my blood boil because there were, and are, much more severe cases than hers. Again, what caused the emotional downturn in this scoliotic woman's life? More on Linda later...

One day, a physical therapist whom I frequently refer clients to and who also has scoliosis, called me to confer over "Simone." Simone was a 14 year-old girl whom we both shared as a client. After working with her for several sessions, the physical therapist mentioned that Simone may benefit from wearing a back brace. Simone's mother was completely unreceptive and dismissed the idea.

Having worked with Simone and having dealt with her mother, I told the therapist that I was pretty sure I knew what was going on – the issues with the brace were more about the mother, than the daughter. For Simone's mom to even consider getting a brace for her daughter would mean admitting that Simone may have a "fault," which can be difficult for a parent. Simone's mother may have been battling the erroneous thought that she was to blame or that her daughter may be "defective."

I use really strong emotional words like "fault" and "defective" in quotations because they are horrendous words to use. But, unfortunately, these are the thoughts that often go through the minds of people who have scoliosis and parents whose children have scoliosis. If these thoughts are, in fact, going through your mind, I urge you to speak to someone about them instead of them bottling up. Speak with your pediatrician or a trusted counselor and let someone help you work through these feelings.

Many varying triggers can add emotional distress, which can complicate one's ability to own his or her scoliosis. While scoliosis is not a personality disorder, it can radically affect how people behave. People living with scoliosis sometimes feel shameful about their condition. The more you own your scoliosis, the less the emotional side of scoliosis will rule your body and mind.

Tread lightly. Get hard, medical data and be aware of the emotional scoliosis card that some people try to play. Scoliosis is 16-dimensional and does not just affect the physical body.

3
embracing your beautiful scolotic back

L ike many others with scoliosis, I have had some very emotionally dark moments. I remember days during intense rehearsals with the Rockettes when certain muscles in my back would seize up and spasm because of my spiral spine. I would be in tremendous pain, but I had to push through for the remaining hours of rehearsal. By the end of the day, I'd be physically and emotionally exhausted. I'd lock myself in my hotel room and wouldn't emerge until the next day's rehearsal started. I'd hear other girls leaving their rooms to go have dinner together or laughing as they went down to socialize with other cast members and I would be so angry that they didn't have my pain. My mother, who wrote a chapter in this book, says she remembers *lots* of tearful phone calls from me during those times.

I needed to choose to be positive and look at the glass as half-full; otherwise, some days felt like my scoliosis would emotionally swallow me whole. My type-A, strong-willed spirit couldn't make my spine totally straight. Believe me, I tried! It was within my power to change my hair style and color, apply my make-up differently, pick a new color of nail polish, change my skin tone by the sun or by self-tanner, choose a different style of clothing, alter my weight by exercise and diet...but I couldn't make my spine straight.

I finally had to make peace with The Lord that exactly how I am is how He chose to beautifully make me. He intimately knows and loves me and He chose me to have this spine. It was a hard pill to swallow, but it gave me such peace. It was a peace that only He could give me. Psalm 119:37 reads, "Your hands made me and fashioned me; give me understanding, that I may learn Your commandments."

Another passage from the Bible that brought peace to my soul was Psalm 139:13-16: "For You formed my inward parts; You wove me in my mother's womb. I will give thanks to You, for I am fearfully and wonderfully made; wonderful are Your works, and my soul knows it very well. My frame was not hidden from You, when I was made in secret, and skillfully wrought in the depths of the earth; Your eyes have seen my unformed substance; and in Your book were all written the days that were ordained for me; when as yet there was not one of them."

Once I made peace with the fact that my spine would never be totally straight and that it was totally out of my control, I started to seek out what I could do for my scoliosis. I had the power to decrease my pain without narcotics or surgery. I also had the power to make sure that the rest of my body wasn't portrayed as sickly. I vowed that I was going to keep my body in the best shape possible to protect my spiral spine. I was not about to let my scoliosis own me and, as God as my witness, I was NOT about to play the scoliosis card. I would never let my scoliosis dictate who I would become. Today, most people don't know I have scoliosis, unless I tell them or show them.

My body is supple and dynamic. It is able to shift and move. Those awesome attributes are my focus. Strength and flexibility are what I hang my scoliotic hat on.

When I work with my clients, we speak a lot about anatomy. Muscle, bone, and fascia are non-emotional topics. I try to give them lots of usable, anatomical knowledge during their lessons. I've found that the more factual, anatomical knowledge a scoliotic person has, the less likely they are to throw scoliotic pity-parties. I want to give them as much power as I can to help them fight this lifelong scoliotic battle. For the scoliotic person, knowledge is power.

Don't get me wrong, though – there is still an emotional battle to fight. I wish that scoliosis was purely physical and that emotions didn't play a part. I find the line between the strictly physical world and the abounding emotional world a hard one to navigate with scoliosis.

Maybe this is why I was so offended when I spoke with my children's former pediatrician about all of my scoliotic endeavors. Early into our conversation, I realized that he was unaware that I had scoliosis, so I simply informed him of my diagnosis. Immediately, his tone became filled with dramatic, unnecessary concern and he sympathetically responded with, "Oh, I'm so sorry." Wait a minute! Scoliosis isn't fatal! His response really ticked me off. I work very hard to educate anyone and everyone that scoliosis is not a death sentence, and it does not have to negatively affect one's quality life. As this battle raged inside my head, I smiled and politely wrapped up our conversation before my double-edged tongue said something I'd regret.

I choose to think that my back is beautiful. Yes, I really do think I have a beautiful back. My bony spine may be a bit spiraled but the muscles around my spine are healthy and beautiful. I look at my achievements and all The Lord has blessed me with and immediately, I am embarrassed that I occasionally fixate on these little curves in my spine.

Some days, having scoliosis is a physical challenge. Other days, it's a mental challenge. When those mentally dark days are looking at you square in the face, I would challenge you to find the beauty in your body. What's your favorite part of your body? Why? What makes your body beautifully different from everyone else's?

I truly believe that an amazing accomplishment in the battle with scoliosis is achieved when you learn to find the beauty in your scoliotic back. This may not happen today or tomorrow, but I promise you that this is an achievable goal. The beauty is there, you just have to look.

4) real life scoliosis stories

Here are a few more interesting stories for you to chew on. I'm sharing these stories with you because I want to illustrate the many ways in which scoliosis can present itself, as well as the different positive and negative ways you can manage it.

"Lana" was an extremely under-conditioned, 60 year-old woman when she first came to see me. Her main curve was in her lumbar spine and was measuring around 50 degrees. No muscles on the right side of her spine even fired for the first few months we worked together. That's how under conditioned her body was. I initially gave her one tiny exercise to do at home, and she ended up in severe muscle spasms.

For the first six months, I had to focus on Lana's overall body strength instead of corrective scoliosis exercises. I'm not going to lie, it was rough and there were a few times I thought I'd lost Lana as a client because her progress was so minimal. Since then, Lana takes two to three Pilates mat classes a week, a private lesson with me every three weeks, followed by a myofascial massage – all to increase her overall bodily strength.

Lana has been a real trooper and wrote these words to me one day:

"In less than a year, I've learned how to begin living in the world of scoliosis. I am more aware now of how I carry myself and how I can counteract the twisting and the sinking into my scoli. I'm stronger to the point that I can do so many more activities that would have sent me into severe back spasms prior to my time with you. My goal is to continue to strengthen my body and to increase my knowledge of scoli so that I can accept and improve where I am and have the quality of life I would like to have."

Lana's story proves that it's never too late to take control and start owning your scoliosis. Pretty cool isn't it? What an inspiration!

"Duke" was the nine year-old grandson of a Pilates teacher that I had trained. His grandma was very worried about his back, so I agreed to work with him and offer my opinion. He obviously had scoliosis, seemingly idiopathic lordosis scoliosis. In the ribcage, we should have a normal vertical curvature going backwards known as kyphosis. In our low backs, we have a normal vertical curve going forwards called lordosis. Yet Duke's upper spine was going forwards, into his chest, instead of backwards. The ribcage lordosis made his spiral spine look worse.

Scoliosis definitely ran in Duke's family, as his mom and other female relatives had it too. The ratio of girls to boys who have spiral spines is roughly 80 to 20, so Duke was in the minority. He was also fairly young to have a curve that looked so spiraled, and have lordosis in his upper back where his scoliosis was.

He hadn't been seen by an orthopedist yet, so I insisted that he go and get X-rays. His major curve was measured in the 30 to 40 degree range and was told to get fitted for a back brace.

Duke *hated* wearing his back brace. He would have huge, screaming arguments with his parents over it. Since insurance didn't cover the cost of an expensive back brace (as it's usually considered "elective" therapy), his grandma graciously offered to pay for it. Unfortunately, Duke's parents felt guilty about the cost of the brace, and it weighed on them heavily. They, in turn, increased the pressure on Duke to wear the brace. Duke didn't budge. Even on vacation at the beach, he not only refused to wear the brace, he wouldn't go into the water or even take his shirt off. He didn't want anyone to see his back.

Over the next few years, I saw Duke just a handful of times. I gave him a few exercises to do and taught his grandma exactly which exercises to work with him on using the Pilates equipment. One day, I drove an hour north to teach him at his grandmother's Pilates studio. I played it cool all lesson to see if he'd open up to me about his back brace and his scoliosis. Sure enough, Duke soon told me how much he hated his brace and just wanted to be like all the other guys. Instinctively, I taught him a few tricks to counteract his scoliosis, even how to look cool by leaning against something when he was hanging out with his friends – no one would ever notice he was actually doing a scoliosis exercise for his back.

As I was getting my stuff together at the end of the lesson, I noticed Duke was slouching in a chair, being cool of course, but he was also actively counteracting his spiral spine. I called him out because I knew what he was doing. He gave me a cool guy grin with a little twinkle in his eye but never mentioned a word.

I *knew* he wanted to help his back…everyone who has scoliosis wants to help his or her back. The key with Duke was figuring out how to connect with him so he'd comply with doing something positive that helped his spiral spine.

"Megan" was in my fifth grade class in elementary school. I remember within that one nine-month school year, Megan's parents chose to put braces on her teeth, get her glasses, and have her fitted for a hard plastic brace for her torso. I realize now the hard plastic brace was for scoliosis. In addition to the braces on her teeth, Megan also had a retainer that fit her top and bottom jaw making it very hard for her to speak and causing her to drool when she spoke up in class. To cover up her full-torso back brace, Megan began wearing big, bulky sweaters. She was a very smart girl, but she had the smallest self-esteem and was very often made fun of in class. Once, a boy put a thumbtack on Megan's chair. She sobbed for over an hour after sitting on that tack. I'm sure there was a bit of physical pain involved, but I think she was crying more over the emotional pain.

I don't know Megan's scoliotic story, so I can't give my two cents on whether a back brace was the best therapy approach. Since you have to see a doctor to get a brace, I must assume that that person deemed the back brace treatment to be the best option for her. Also, I can understand getting fitted for glasses so she could see, but what troubles me is adding braces for her teeth including a double jaw retainer in the same year! My father is a dentist, as is my father-in-law. I've been in the dental world my whole life. I had braces and headgear for three years in middle school and I know what a child goes through emotionally. Could the orthodontic work have been held off for a few years? Was the orthodontic work a medical necessity or was it for vanity reasons?

Parents, please carefully consider how many new medical treatments you put your scoliotic child through in one year.

"Jane" came to me one year after having scoliotic spinal surgery. She had a spinal fusion from T3 to S1 (slightly below her neck down into her pelvis) in her mid-50s. A year had passed but she was still dealing with back pain. Jane had gone back to her surgeon because of it and he suggested she try Pilates. For the following three years, she diligently attended two Pilates group Reformer classes every week to manage her pain.

Jane was a wonderful client to work with, but I always wondered if her spinal fusion was necessary. Again, I'm not a surgeon so I have to trust that the surgeon deemed it so. What caused me to question the necessity was when Jane told me her surgeon chose to do the surgery "because he didn't want my scoliosis to get worse." She never told me what, if any, decrease in curvature was achieved. A surgery like that can never be reversed, so I chose to never open that door with Jane. She still had quite a kyphotic curve in her upper back (a rounded forward spine), which was not scoliosis related. Her back was fused in that kyphotic position which caused chronic neck problems for Jane. All I could do for her was emotionally encourage her, stabilize the fused portion of her body with muscles that weren't cut and injured in her spinal fusion surgery, and mobilize and stabilize the movable portions of her body. I always wondered if Jane could have avoided her spinal fusion had she been redirected to Pilates to manage her scoliosis prior to surgery. We'll never know.

"Georgia" was a 17-year-old woman when her emotionally-exhausted mom called me. Her mom read the first edition of *The Beautiful Scoliotic Back* and realized she lived in the same town as I did and wanted to know if I could help her daughter.

After an hour-long phone conversation with Georgia's mother, I learned her daughter had pulled herself out of a prestigious private school in town to be homeschooled, despite the fact that her parents didn't approve of the decision and her younger sister was still attending that school. Georgia also announced she wanted spinal fusion surgery and the date was set up for two months from when her mom initially called me. I bluntly asked her mom how her marriage was doing from all this and that's when the floodgates opened. She shared that this emotional stress was tearing the entire family apart, including her marriage. Georgia was such a pretty girl but had so much shame about her back and openly blamed her parents. Her parents were not equipped to handle all that Georgia's spiral spine was dishing out.

I agreed to see her daughter the next week. I told her mom that I wasn't promising miracles with her back, but did say that movement can have a profound affect on the human body. I told her that at this point, my goal was to help Georgia make peace with her scoliosis. I wanted, I *needed*, her to not make this decision rashly, but with a sound mind.

After Georgia blew off several lessons, I left her a very long voicemail telling her I would love to just have a conversation with her. I prayed that she would have peace with her scoliosis and peace about surgery. I asked her to not make a rash decision she'd later regret. Amazingly, two weeks later my phone rang and I saw Georgia's name come up. I quickly answered the phone, but no one replied and then the call was dropped. I immediately called Georgia back but she didn't pick up, so I left a message. Twenty minutes went by when I finally got a call back. All Georgia said was, "I'm sorry, I accidently butt-dialed you." She gracefully said goodbye and hung up the phone. That was it.

My heart ached for Georgia. I wondered how many times throughout that two week time period she had listened to my long voice message. She had obviously already made up her mind at this point, so all I could do was pray for her.

I heard through the grapevine that Georgia had surgery and is happy. Her spine is perfectly straight and she loves it. When the emotional side of scoliosis takes over all other realms of life, I think that may be a rare time when surgery might be a good option. The emotional scars of scoliosis rip deeply through the hearts of the entire family. I hope those scars get tended to someday for Georgia and her family. Those deep scars usually last a lifetime.

"Nancy" is a precious client of mine whom I've worked with for years. Nancy is about 60 years-old, but has taken such good care of herself that she looks and acts like a 40 year-old. She holds a nursing degree and is very knowledgeable about the human body. This client is such an inspiration, especially because of the bodily drama she's battled for years.

When I first started working with Nancy, she suffered from debilitating migraines multiple times a week and had a pretty motionless scoliotic spine. It is typical of a person who has had spinal fusion surgery to have an immobile spine, but Nancy hadn't had that surgery to straighten out her scoliosis. Why, then, was her spine motionless?

Many body practitioners had tried every trick in the scoliosis book to ease the tightness in Nancy's "scoliotic" back. She finally decided to have an X-ray taken to determine her back's degree of curvature. Lo and behold, her scoliosis was diagnosed as mild, since it was less than 10 degrees. Scoliosis is a lateral curve of the spine and the medical community considers 10 degrees to be the minimum degree marker for a diagnosis of scoliosis.

Her spine and body acted very scoliotic, but there were many other contributing factors, which funneled into her body causing it to act the way it did. Scoliosis was not the main culprit in Nancy's case. I believe the main culprit was the 20-plus years of her multi-week migraines that triggered her back muscles to continually seize up.

Nancy devoutly sticks to her schedule of a weekly private GYROTONIC® lesson with me, a weekly Pilates private, a weekly restorative yoga group class, and an alternating bi-weekly massage between a myofascial therapist and a neuromuscular therapist. She also sees a physical therapist when needed.

Recently, Nancy purchased a Pilates Reformer and Tower along with a Pilates Chair to keep her body working well at home. Her schedule will be changing slightly because she'll be taking care of her two grandbaby boys a few days a week and is anticipating her spine throwing a bit of a fit. Nancy's dedication to her bodily health is admirable.

Simone, whom I mentioned earlier in the book, has a happy ending to her story, despite how her emotional scoliosis story began. Her mother finally pulled her head out of the sand and realized that her daughter's back needed special attention.

Amazingly, Simone had never had an X-ray to determine the degree of her curves, despite seeing a physical therapist who suggested she get fitted for a brace. I insisted she get an X-ray to develop a baseline for her scoliosis. Simone's very first X-ray showed that her major curve was measuring just below 50 degrees. Why Simone's scoliosis wasn't caught before this point was beyond me – especially because she was such a dedicated ballet dancer and spent hours each day in a leotard and tights standing in front of a mirror. And to top it off, her mom homeschooled her.

A brace was immediately prescribed by her new orthopedic surgeon, which she wore devoutly because she now started to see and understand the magnitude of her spiral spine. She started to own her scoliosis.

During the six months that I worked with Simone, I encouraged her and her mom to do as much research as possible. I'd give them some leads on research and they'd run with them. Soon, they were off to their first Curvy Girls conference. Curvy Girls is a national organization that helps girls with scoliosis lead support groups for other girls living with scoliosis in their hometowns. Simone came back energized and more at peace with her scoliosis.

Fortunately, during that time Simone came to the realization on her own that ballet was hurting, not helping her spiral spine and decided to quit cold turkey. I encouraged the decision despite her mom's hesitancy.

Unfortunately, none of the work I was doing with Simone was showing the results I wanted. Simone's curve increased. It was time to call in the reinforcements. Happily, both mother and daughter were ready to deal with scoliosis head on. From another lead I gave them, they went up to Wisconsin for a two-week Schroth physical therapy intensive program.

I don't see Simone anymore for lessons because she dutifully performs her daily, hour-long Schroth exercises on her own as prescribed by her Schroth physical therapists. I'm so grateful Simone's and her mother's eyes were opened and Simone started owning her scoliosis. I just wonder if all this running around and quick decision-making would've been needed if they had dealt with Simone's scoliosis when they first saw it.

"Elizabeth" came to see me after her regular Pilates instructor called me stumped and confused as to what was going on with Elizabeth's back. That should have been my first red flag. This particular instructor used to work for me, was a former professional ballet dancer and thoroughly understood the human body. She also had a very sharp mind and was a phenomenal Pilates instructor - a rare breed. This instructor informed me that her client had scoliosis and was in acute pain from it. I agreed to work with Elizabeth in an attempt to sort out this befuddling bodily puzzle for this 50 year-old client.

Sure enough, Elizabeth had moderate scoliosis in stereotypical fashion. I think her major curve was measuring in the 30 to 40 degree area. Her scoliosis made sense to me, but her odd sacral pain did not. I was able to map out her scoliosis, but there were red flags concerning her lumbar and sacral areas. I agreed to continue working with her, but strongly suggested she see a physical therapist to check out her lumbar spine. The visit with the physical therapist led to an MRI, which led to the discovery of a very large cyst inside her spinal canal that was pushing on her spinal chord.

Neither Elizabeth nor I were huge advocates of back surgery, but we both knew this was different. Within two weeks, she had surgery to remove the spinal cyst, yet she chose to leave her spiral spine untouched. Within a few weeks, she was back to her regular, multi-weekly Pilates sessions with her normal Pilates instructor and her sacral pain had subsided.

Like Elizabeth, if your attempt to own your scoliosis doesn't line up with the knowledge you've acquired, there may be a deeper underlying cause to your pain.

"Sarah" and "Kaitlin" are genetically identical twins and both have idiopathic scoliosis. Interestingly, their scoliosis presents

30

itself very differently. I started working with them when they were 11 years-old, right after they were diagnosed with scoliosis.

Kaitlin had open-heart surgery at birth and was smaller in height, weight, and build from Sarah. Kaitlin's main curve is in her upper thoracic spine and goes to the right, away from the heart that was operated on upon birth. Sarah's curve is more balanced between her thoracic and lumbar curves.

Within a four-month time period of bi-weekly and shared semi-private lesson between the two girls, their spines both changed. Sarah's thoracic curve went from 15 degrees down to 13 degrees and her lumbar curve went from 15 degrees down to 8 degree. Sarah's mom told me that upon measuring the new X-ray, the orthopedist said, "I never see anyone reverse their curves and get better." Well, there's a first time for everything, Doc.

Kaitlin's back was a bit of a different story. Her thoracic curve had increased from 10 degrees to 15 degrees, but her lumbar curve had decreased from 10 degrees to zero degrees. I was actually discouraged by this as I wanted to keep a curve in her lumbar spine in order to balance the curve in her thoracic spine. As a rule with scoliosis, it's preferable to have a bit of a curve in the top and in the bottom of the spine, so that they balance each other out. Kaitlin's body was responding to movement and exercise, but I suspected her heart surgery was the root cause of the issue I was having with the top curve.

I sent Kaitlin to my favorite myofascial therapist to work on her rounded forward shoulders and upper right thoracic curve. I suspected there was some deep scar tissue and bound fascia from her heart surgery at birth. After the massage, her shoulders "dis-attached" from her sternum, the area that was cut open for her surgery over 11 years ago. Six months later,

Kaitlin's next X-ray showed her upper curve had stabilized at 15 degrees and her bottom curve was now back to stabilize her top, settling at 14 degrees.

Throughout that same six-month time period, Sarah had gotten braces for her teeth and headgear to correct an overbite. Her mom and I had many long conversations where I conveyed my fears of orthodontic work for people with scoliosis. Her mom understood everything I was telling her but decided to risk it and get the braces anyways. Sarah also broke her right wrist two weeks before her X-rays. With all those changes to her body, I was amazed that her top curve only progressed to 17 degrees. Happily, her lower curve stayed put at eight degrees.

The twins just had new X-rays and despite both girls having phenomenal growth spurts in the last few months, both girls' scoliosis curves decreased. Sarah's curves are measuring at 10 degrees in her thoracic curve and zero degrees in her lumbar curve. Happily her last six months have been free of new orthodontic work and a broken arm, which I think had a lot to do with her curves increasing at the last X-rays. Kaitlin's back has stabilized at 14 degrees in her thoracic curve and 11 degrees in lumbar curve.

The orthopedist said "they're just lucky" and wasn't interested in their mom telling him what they've proactively been doing for their spiral spines. Even if their orthopedist hasn't seen the light with proactive corrective exercise, their mom has.

"Ted." I only worked with Ted once, and he was clearly looking for a miracle fix, which I was unable to give him. I wish I had a picture to show you of this 60-something-year-old man. Just know that my words will never give you the full picture of Ted's body.

If you were looking at Ted from the front, he noticeably had one shoulder higher than the other with a rib-shift going in that same direction, to the right. His pelvis jutted out sideways to the left and his knees laterally jutted out in the opposite direction, to the right (stand up and try putting yourself in that position – it hurts). I'm not kidding you, when he stepped into the Pilates studio I stared at this man's body in disbelief.

His scoliosis was much lower in his back than the norm. His knees were what baffled me, though. Knees are supposed to bend forward and backward, but for some reason both of his knees were bending to the right. Because I couldn't put all the puzzle pieces of his body together right away, I decided to get him moving on a piece of Pilates equipment so I could watch his body in action.

It took him a full two minutes to simply lie-down on the machine. His entire body was so bound up. My body ached just watching Ted move. It was quite apparent he hadn't taken very good care of himself over his lifetime and I remember thinking he wasn't old enough to be moving that way. I'd seen 80 year-olds move better than he was moving.

As the lesson progressed, it dawned on me that Ted's scoliosis had gone down into his knees. When there is an "S" curve in the back, there is the main curve (usually at the top) and then a compensatory curve (usually a little lower down in the spine), so the person doesn't walk around in a side-bend. Well, Ted's main curve happened so low in his spine that I'm very certain his knees took the job of being the secondary compensating curve. The knees were the next joint down the bony chain that could move and compensate for the main curve in his spine and pelvis.

I picked Ted's brain throughout the lesson on his health story and the man had a zillion surgeries done on his body...but not one done on his spiral spine. He never fixed the real problem, which was his scoliosis. He fixed all the little pains that happened on his appendages, but not the problem itself. I found it interesting that no orthopedist had intervened to suggest to him what the main issue was.

The last I heard about Ted, he'd had another knee surgery. A few months afterward, his scoliosis had gotten much worse. At that time, Ted was considering filing a lawsuit against the knee surgeon claiming the surgery made his scoliosis worse.

In my opinion, Ted never owned his scoliosis and was therefore the victim of a medical community, which didn't fully understand his scoliosis either. He had been reactive instead of proactive. Throughout his lifetime, he shifted the blame from one surgeon to another. Ted complained about the cost of pre-hab (a fun word I use that is short for pre-habilitation). If you do pre-hab, it'll most likely keep you from doing re-hab, rehabilitation after a surgery. Aren't medical bills expensive? What if you shifted the money around and paid that money in the beginning so you never had to pay it at the end to have surgery?

The moral of the story with Ted is that you need to learn to own your scoliosis. Don't put the full responsibility for your scoliosis in anyone else's hands. Weigh everyone's advice, including physicians'. Learn to own and manage the spine you've been given.

Linda, whom I mentioned earlier, was a pro at playing the scoliosis card. About six years after I initially worked with her at my big Pilates studio, she saw me for a lesson at my private studio. She was now in her mid-30s. I was stunned when the lesson was booked. I thought she was too far-gone mentally to want to get proactive help for her scoliosis.

Since I'd seen her last, Linda had some sort of neurological implant inserted under her skin on her spine to help manage her pain. She was still in a lot of pain though, so I didn't know if it was doing any good. Muscles on one side of her near 50-degree lumbar spiral spine were so overbuilt and beefy that it made her lumbar "hump" look very pronounced. Muscles on the other side of her extremely concaved back didn't fire at all.

She referred to her lower back muscular protrusion as "it" and was amazed that I would touch "it" while cuing her in different exercises. She told me that if she ever gets married she'd have her veil go far enough down her back so "it" was covered. Linda only wore black shirts "because black covers up everything." She made other negative comments about herself, blaming everything on her scoliosis, which made it very obvious that I needed to spend time loving on her soul while I worked on her back.

She was a bright woman. Remember, she was pre-med in college. I intricately began talking about what was happening in different systems of her body due to her spiral spine and we would discuss it all lesson. I took all emotion out of these conversations and just talked facts.

She'd been having severe lumbar/sacral pain for a few years and was considering getting her bottom two vertebras fused. After working with her for a while, I realized that her scoliosis went down through her pelvis into her knees. I told her I was pretty sure that fusing just two vertebra would only put her back into surgery once again in a few more years because it would have ticked her scoliosis off just enough to increase the curve somewhere else.

We openly talked about the basic idea behind spinal fusion surgery, which was to stabilize an unstable spine. Since her major curve was over 40 degrees, she was a candidate for it. The goal of surgery would be to decrease the degree of curvature. Surgery is often done with a combination of rods, screws, hooks, and bone grafts that fuse the affected scoliotic vertebrae together. Linda understood everything we discussed.

Next, she started meeting with different surgeons, diligently trying to find the right one. One day, I noticed that her inquiries to doctors had stopped and I asked why. She very astutely said, "I think getting surgery done by the wrong surgeon is worse than not having surgery." I absolutely agreed with her but was amazed at what I had heard (she was really owning her scoliosis!). She felt like some of these surgeons knew how to deal with her facet issue, or knew how to deal with her stenosis issue, but not all under the major umbrella of her scoliosis. After much discussion, I suggested she try to get an appointment with a pediatric orthopedist who specialized in scoliosis. Finding a surgeon who specialized in scoliosis for adults seemed to be quite challenging.

As I've stated previously, I am rarely an advocate for surgery, but there are always exceptions. In Linda's case, surgery was already imminent. I encouraged her to talk to the surgeon about fusing her lower curve, in addition to the double vertebra fusion for her stenosis. Her upper curve was beautifully mobile and barely affected her shoulder girdle. We talked about it for weeks and she too, came to the conclusion that this was the right path to take. Psychologically, her "hump" would be gone from her life.

Emotionally, Linda was still in agony. I spoke to many of her family members, looking for guidance and clues from her past as to how I could emotionally connect with her. One family member reiterated to me that Linda had been a three-time varsity athlete, awarded college scholarships, had a beautiful face, and always had so much going for her. It was shame over her back that had Linda distraught with her life.

One day I decided it was time to open up the fears that were encased by her scoliosis. No joke, with the very first word that came out of her mouth, her eyes teared up and her bottom lip started to quiver. Linda blurted out, "My deepest desire is to have a baby and play tennis. I also want a career but...," scoliosis was the crux of every single issue she spoke about. The floodgates had been opened and she emoted non-stop for 20 minutes. Every single fear was absolutely legitimate. She had just let the fears envelope her like a cocoon and hadn't spoken to anyone about them.

She feared her spiral spine would inhibit her from having a baby. I told her that my body handled it just fine and I've also worked with pregnant scoli clients who had more of a degree than I did, and they were fine, too. I've even worked with pregnant ladies who'd had scoliosis spinal fusion surgery prior to getting pregnant and they were fine, but did have to have a C-section.

Amazingly, that old athlete was still in her, and it was dying to come out. She had previously decided that tennis would be the best sport for her because she didn't have to have a team for it. She worried, however, that her body wouldn't be able to handle tennis. We went down the list of her fears one at a time. I gave her real life stories of how others had handled those same fears and backed them up by medical research.

A few months after successfully working with Linda, a family member texted me the following: "(Linda) said she was going to go to Home Depot to buy a dowel (to do some scoliosis exercises). I almost drove off the road. #miracleworker." Another text a month later read, "(another family member) thinks she's getting way more than back therapy from you. You're so good for her confidence."

Not everything in the scoliosis world is black and white. Actually, I would say everything is gray when dealing with spiral spines. Be sure and look at all of the dimensions of scoliosis when working with someone who has a spiral spine.

"Tina" was a 40-something-year-old, stay-at-home mother of five children, ranging from a kindergartener to teenagers. She emailed me and said she was looking for someone who could help her manage her scoliosis to help with her chronic lower back pain.

After our first lesson, it was pretty obvious that her weak core (from birthing five children) and her major 30 to 40 degree scoliosis curve in her lumbar spine was causing her constant state of pain.

We had a lesson every few weeks and she was extremely attentive, wanting to thoroughly understand the intricacies of her scoliosis. I gave her exercises to do at home and taught her how to myofascially release certain muscles in her back by using some small balls. She texted me one day saying she hadn't had back pain in a week. A few exercises, some knowledge of her back, and a few plastic balls seemed to do the trick.

Tina read the first edition of *The Beautiful Scoliotic Back* and spoke to her mom about it. Her mom opened up to Tina and told her how much she had worried about her back, and had from the first time she was diagnosed so many years ago. Her mom said she was so relieved Tina was working on her scoliosis. Until then, Tina had no idea how her mom had struggled with those thoughts and was so grateful she had talked to her.

"Joy" reminded me of Tiny Tim from *A Christmas Carol*. At the age of 12, she looked malnourished, and to be very blunt, crippled. I could write an entire book on my yearlong experience with Joy, but I'll condense it here.

Joy's mother died about five years earlier and her dad was a deadbeat. Joy, along with 11 other brothers, sisters, and cousins, lived with her grandmother and her grandmother's two sisters in one house. I heard about this hot mess of a situation through a client and agreed to work on Joy's scoliotic body.

Her body didn't make sense to me. Obviously, there was scoliosis, but there was so much more that wasn't adding up. To top it off, Joy's emotional intelligence was very low. She'd had so much emotional trauma in her short life that she couldn't mentally focus on the intricacies of her body. There was no mind-body movement connection. All she wanted was to have fun and be loved on by me.

I called her grandma after the lesson, as a family friend had brought her to the lesson, and asked her what the doctors had said about Joy's body. I was then informed she hadn't been to the doctor since her mom passed away. Sigh. The grandma then informed me that I was welcome to take Joy to the doctor. Me? At first, I was floored that she would suggest I bring her, but after I thought about it, who else would? Who was there to tend to Joy's spiral spine's health? After I spent some time with the Lord, I agreed.

I picked up Joy and her grandma and off we went to the best orthopedist in town, whom I'd scheduled Joy an appointment with shortly after our first lesson. It didn't take long for me to figure out that Joy's grandma was illiterate. I knew then that I was the one who would be talking with the orthopedist and making sense of Joy's body. It turns out that Joy had a five-centimeter leg length discrepancy, meaning part of her scoliosis was functional. She also had a hemi vertebra, which is when a bone is misshapen, looking more like a triangle than a square.

The spine, therefore, does not sit straight above or below that misshapen vertebra. As if that wasn't enough, she was genetically missing five vertebra and some of the vertebra she did have were genetically fused in the wrong places. These issues are often put in the category of congenital scoliosis, where aspects of the spine are not fully formed, or malformed, in utero.

A lot went on during the next nine months, including multiple platform shoes fitted for Joy, lots of doctor's visits, more X-rays, and a CT Scan. At this point, it was very obvious, for many reasons, that she needed surgery. Her scoliosis was worsening, as was her bodily pain. Some of her bones were misshapen, but proper exercise couldn't change the shape of bone, only surgery could.

I was there for Joy's nine-hour surgery and visited her every day in the hospital. To say it was horrible is an understatement. She had to have a blood transfusion a few days after surgery, and the nausea and pain overwhelmed her. Her grandmother didn't care for her one lick in the hospital, so it was my good friend and I that did. I was there when she had to learn how to walk again with the physical therapist in the hospital and for many other recovery milestones.

The yearlong journey ending in surgery for Joy, truly altered my life and how I view scoliosis surgery. Is there a time and a place for spinal fusion surgery? Yes. But, after you've seen the immediate aftermath of two stainless steel rods and 17 screws drilled into a girl's back like a Home Depot commercial, it breaks your heart and brings you to your knees. Or, the month-long housebound seclusion after the surgery when Joy became addicted to prescribed pain meds for her unbelievably immense pain – it's enough to change a woman for life. I can't blame Joy for her addiction, because all of the systems of her body (muscular, bony, fascial, nervous, organ, circular, etc.) had been living in that crooked position for 12 years, and in a matter of nine hours, all those systems were yanked, drilled, sawed, and screwed into a 45-degree different angle. Her entire body was in *massive* overload and no one was there to love on her during her long recovery.

While she was in the hospital, I felt compelled to bring her one of my young son's baby blankets. At the age of 12, the only things Joy wanted me to do for her was to tuck her in with the two-by-two foot blanket, rub the blue satin fabric corner on her cheek, and sing to her.

After serving Joy for over a year, I would never wish spinal fusion surgery on a soul, but Joy had no other option. She needed the surgery. Does everyone who has scoliosis need to go through scoliosis spinal fusion surgery? The answer is unequivocally no.

If you have tried every other option out there for your back and think your only option is surgery, please serve someone who is currently going through the surgery. Serve someone immediately after the surgery while still in the hospital, a month after surgery, a year after surgery, ten years after surgery. Intimately know what you are getting yourself into. It will change your life. Then, and only then, do you have enough knowledge to make the huge decision as to whether to have scoliosis spinal fusion surgery.

After you thoroughly know what you are getting yourself into and decide surgery is your correct path, find the most experienced orthopedic surgeon specializing in scoliosis you can find. Joy's surgeon was amazing. He was the most senior surgeon I could get my hands on and he had plenty of gray-haired wisdom to match it. With all of her bodily issues he was doing surgery on, he could have easily left her a paraplegic from the operation. He was very upfront with me and told me Joy could have neurological issues after the surgery. Happily, none of that came into fruition.

There is a light at the end of the story for Joy. Despite her grandmother not bringing her to one of the multiple physical therapy appointments I set up post-surgery, Joy is doing amazingly well. She has a glow in her eyes I'd never seen before. Her leg length discrepancy is down to 1.5 centimeters and her back looks wonderful. Joy looks like a normal kid. She's finally growing and she can keep up with all her brothers, sisters, and cousins in that hot mess of a house she's living in. Her most prized accomplishment is that she can ride a bike, which she had never been able to do prior to surgery. Joy asked for a bike for Christmas.

Naomi, mentioned earlier in the book, was diagnosed at the age of seven with a 17-degree scoliotic curve. Her pediatrician found her scoliosis when she went in for a routine yearly physical. Both of Naomi's parents are esteemed professors at a prestigious university and were worried about Naomi's back. They did their research and found a good pediatric orthopedic surgeon in town who saw Naomi every six months for check-ups.

Soon after she was diagnosed, Naomi's parents not only began taking her to weekly Iyengar yoga lessons, they also started her on a regimen of physical therapy. At that point, Naomi also began visiting a myofascial massage therapist. Within the year, the curve improved – falling to 12 degrees.

When she was nine years old, her curve jumped to 23 degrees. Naomi's mom thinks this mostly had to do with Naomi beginning her pubescent growth spurt. Around that time, Naomi started seeing me regularly for Pilates lessons.

I set a strict schedule for Naomi, doing one Pilates Mat group class and one Pilates Reformer group class with me every week. About every three weeks, Naomi also had a corrective private Pilates lesson with me.

One day, Naomi's rather stoic father came in to my studio to pick Naomi up from Pilates class – a day I will never forget. He was holding Naomi's newest back X-rays in his hands and tears were in his eyes. Within the first six months of doing Pilates with me, the curve in Naomi's spine had decreased by five degrees. Her curve was back down to 17 degrees. Naomi's parents realized that everyday activities could possibly negatively affect their daughter's scoliosis, so they carefully assessed every decision as it came. In fifth grade, it was time for Naomi to pick which musical instrument to play. After a Pilates lesson one day, we all sat together and analyzed which instrument would be best (and worst) for her scoliosis. After all the biomechanics of holding the instruments were carefully considered, we voted on the clarinet to be the winner.

Throughout the years, Naomi's scoliotic curvature has toggled up and down a few degrees relative to her growth spurts. Naomi's parents have also changed her scoliotic regimen to deal with the circumstances at hand. I remember a three-month period in which Naomi was out of the country with her parents. Naomi had to manage her own scoliosis with a routine of exercises and stretches I had set for her. It was a great period of mental growth for Naomi because she was forced to own her scoliosis during that time. When she felt like she was having a twisted day, she had to figure out how to stretch herself out because there was no one there to help her.

When one exercise regimen seemed to stop producing results, Naomi's parents would try another. Naomi is now a 16-year-old beautiful and smart young woman. Both lower and upper curves are tracking at around 13 degrees, which they have remained at for about the last three years. Her orthopedic surgeon said he'd release her next year from yearly check-ups if this trend continues.

Today, Naomi's scoliotic regimen is a blend of multiple exercise forms and bodily practitioners: one weekly private lesson focused on GYROTONIC® exercises with me, one weekly yoga lesson, one weekly Pilates group class (either Mat or Reformer), and a myofascial massage every month. Over the last year her mom started bringing her to acupuncture for menstrual issues and found it had a profound affect on her back. Naomi also has a monthly acupuncture appointment, or goes whenever she needs extra help unwinding her spiral spine.

Naomi's mom's general feeling is that the core strengthening provided by Pilates and GYROTONIC® exercises has been the most useful for stabilizing Naomi's curve, even more so than yoga or massage. Naomi's parents jumped in with both feet to see if different bodily techniques would help Naomi's back and, fortunately, they did!

One day, Naomi's mom and I chatted about all that Naomi was doing for her body. Her mom profoundly told me that all these things are good for overall health, regardless if one has scoliosis or not. I had to sit back and admire her mom's view on committing to her daughter's bodily health.

By no means am I saying I'm a miracle worker or that this solution will work for everyone. Truth be told, I had no clue what I was doing when I started working with Naomi, who was my first scoliosis client. I truly lived up to the old adage of "fake it til you make it." I had great Pilates training and knew how to align a body, and that's how I started with Naomi. Well-trained Pilates professionals specialize in correct alignment. Obviously,

I gained a ton of knowledge throughout the next few years, but in the beginning, I was a well-trained Pilates instructor – and I was able to decrease Naomi's curve. If you can find a well-trained Pilates instructor in your town, that's a wonderful place to start.

Every scoliotic body is different and needs to be treated with individual care. I simply wanted to illustrate how hard Naomi's parents fought, and continue to fight, for their daughter and her scoliotic back. Recently, we've been talking about college with Naomi, and her mom is quite firm that the town her college will be in has to be large enough for at least one Pilates studio.

I will openly say that Naomi and her parents have a special place in my heart. I wish more parents were willing to sift through all the scoliotic data and not give up on their child's body. Naomi's mom wrote this wonderful note to me after I asked her to double-check all my facts on Naomi's scoliotic story:

"You have a very special place in our hearts too! What's been so important to me is to see not only how you've helped 'Naomi's' curve, but more importantly, how you've helped her to understand and take command over her own body. You are always so positive with her (and with me!). So thank you!"

As you can see, spiral spines come in all different shapes and sizes. Scoliosis affects each person's body and mind differently. Now I hope it's understandable why I refer to scoliosis as 16-dimensional. There isn't a one-size-fits-all approach to all the spiral spine stories I just shared with you.

Once scoliosis becomes part of your life, or your family's life, start doing your research. Get X-rays. Talk to as many people as you can from different professions, all of whom will have different takes on how to deal with scoliosis. Try different exercise forms and body practitioners. Settle on a proactive routine that works for you and your body, but be willing to change courses if the outcomes are not as you please. Find someone you can emotionally confide in. Make peace with your body. It's about the journey, not the end goal. Enjoy the journey!

5)

navigating the medical world

I will never have spinal fusion surgery for my scoliosis, so I find it silly to subject myself to radiation from X-rays every year. The X-rays wouldn't change how I'm dealing with my scoliosis. However, I wanted to include X-rays of my back in this book to show everyone what scoliosis looks like, and prevent you from being shocked when you go into the orthopedist for the first time and see the X-ray of your own spiral spine.

I called my one-and-only pediatrician in Minnesota to get copies of the initial X-rays that were taken when I was 14 years-old. These were the only childhood X-rays I had ever had. Lo and behold, the practice had discarded my entire patient file. Eighteen years of my life – gone. My parents hadn't thought to get a copy of my scoliosis X-rays at the time, so those were gone as well. I now know that it's common practice for files to be discarded after a number of years. I would recommend that you get copies of everything and keep your own file up-to-date.

So, now I needed to schedule an appointment with an orthopedist to get X-rays taken. I was a bit curious as to where my curve was measuring, since I'd had two kids. My hormones have been all over the place for a few years, which I know affects a scoliotic spine.

I just needed a spinal X-ray, that's it. After waiting for over a half-hour in the orthopedist's waiting room for my scheduled appointment, I was finally ushered into the X-ray room. The technician told me that the only metal I needed to remove was my belt, which seemed odd. During my X-ray, I asked the technician if I could get an additional X-ray of my rib rotation so I could get a baseline for that measurement. She said they don't normally do that, which means I'd have to rely on my scoliometer for that. A scoliometer is a simple device that looks like a rounded level used to roughly determine the degree of rotation in the scoliotic back. It's about the size of an adult's stretched-out hand. Body practitioners can measure clients' backs with this before and after lessons to see if a decrease in vertebral rotation has been achieved during the lesson.

While leaving the X-ray room, I asked for a copy of the X-rays for my records. The woman obliged and few minutes later, I walked back to my room, X-rays in hand, to wait for the orthopedist. After I was back in the room by myself, I flipped on the X-ray light board, threw my X-rays up and steam started spewing out my ears. I was only given a portion of my full back X-ray. My entire major scoliotic curve wasn't even fully shown on my X-ray. *Argh!*

On top of that, all the metal in my bra, my cross necklace, buttons on my sweater, and metal on my jeans were jumbling up my back X-ray. The metal won't necessarily affect an orthopedist from measuring my Cobb Angle, but it would affect a body practitioner from seeing a macro picture of what's happening in my spine.

The orthopedist finally came in and he unfolded his X-ray, which was three-times longer than my X-ray copy. After looking at it on the X-ray light board, he said, "Well, you have scoliosis, but it's a mild case. It looks like your curve is in the upper 20s or lower 30s." For the record, that's not a *mild* case. I asked him what my exact Cobb Angle measurement was and he seemed shocked that I asked. He said, "Well, I'll have to measure that. If you give me your cell phone number, I'll call you by the end of the week with the measurement." So, at this point I had received no exact Cobb Angle measurement, no full spine X-ray, and no rotational degree measurement. This orthopedist was not helping me own my scoliosis!

I asked him if I could get a copy of the full spine X-ray and he said, "Well, my technician is busy right now and is only here on Tuesdays and Thursdays." Undeterred, I said, "Could you mail them to me?" He wiggled the X-ray to show me how flimsy it was (thank you very much sir, I've seen one or two X-rays) and said, "X-rays are too flimsy to mail." Now, I know for a fact that X-rays are shipped all around the world on a daily basis. But, instead of arguing, I said, "Well, could I come back to the office to pick them up on a later day?" He finally agreed to that. Mind you, if this doctor had more up-to-date equipment, the X-rays would have been digital. He could have printed me a copy, emailed me the document, or scanned a CD with the images on them.

Now, back to the "upper 20s or lower 30s" comment on my current scoliotic curve. That totally freaked me out because that's MORE THAN a 10-degree increase since I last had my X-ray taken at the age of 14...and it totally didn't concern the orthopedist. He said that scoliosis usually increases one to two degrees a year. I've read the medical journals and have done my fair share of research and that doesn't usually start to happen until the age of 50 or you reach a 40-degree curve. I didn't match either of those criteria.

Let's just guess I had a 28-degree curve (and I'm going on the very low end of what the doc said my curve may be at). If a two-degree increase happened annually, I'd have a 72-degree curve by the time I was 50. It'd be a 172-degree curve if I lived to be 100. Let's be a little bit more conservative and say I only experienced a one-degree curve increase each year. At the age of 50, my spine would be at a 50-degree curve and at 100, my curve would be at a 100-degree curve...ain't no way, Doc!

I think the doctor must have noticed my eyes bulge out of my head at his comment because he said, "You're right on track as to where your scoliosis should be." How could he know that without more extensive analysis of my spine, comparative evaluations from my history, and especially without measuring my exact Cobb Angle?

He asked me if I was having any neurological pain and I said no. He still wanted to tap his little hammer on my knees and ankles to make sure they were working fine. Yep, reflexes still look good.

He said I just needed to come back in two to three years to check in and get another X-ray to see if my back was bad enough for surgery at that time. Lovely. He gave me no physical therapy referral – nothing. No Doc, you may not book me for scoliosis surgery. Once again, I was reminded that not all orthopedists are created equal in regards to caring for someone with scoliosis.

The following Friday, I received the promised phone call from the orthopedist. My major curve was measuring at 31 degrees and my compensatory curve was measuring at 23 degrees. That was a hard phone call for me to receive. That Friday was an emotionally dark day for me. My major curve was on the more liberal end of his original guess, not the conservative end.

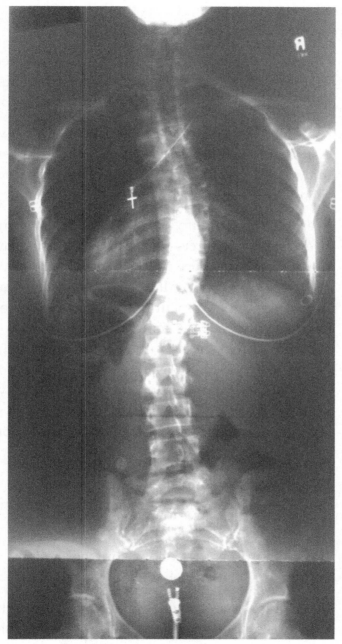

The orthopedist's X-ray of my back.

Based on my experience, I've compiled a few suggestions to help you prepare for your scoliosis X-rays:

- Go to a non-surgical orthopedist or an orthopedist that specializes in scoliosis. The last orthopedist I saw was a spine specialist but didn't specifically specialize in scoliosis.

- Ask the orthopedist in advance if rotational X-rays and measurements can be taken. This can be achieved many different ways.

- Wear a sports bra (if you are female and old enough to need one) and exercise pants that don't have any metal on them in case a gown isn't offered to you by the X-ray technician. All the metal in your X-rays may hinder your body practitioners' ability to correctly analyze your scoliotic spine. Also, I want to point out that the doctor works for the patient and you have the right to tell the doctor exactly what you want out of the exam and X-rays. If you are going to own your scoliosis, you need to speak up, ask for what you want, and not just settle for what is usually done.

- Schedule your X-rays in the morning. Studies have shown that early morning X-rays have lower Cobb Angle measurements than those taken later in the day.

- If possible, do your scoliotic stretches and exercises beforehand if you are having a bound day.

- If possible, have a myofascial massage the night before to unlock your ribcage. This may also show a decrease in curvature on your X-ray. The goal is to not falsely decrease your Cobb Angle by doing some of the above suggestions, but to simply see if your spine is still malleable and able to change. You may reach a point where those things will make no difference in your Cobb Angle.

Now, I will try any form of therapy once to see if it will positively affect my scoliosis. I was hesitant, but I sucked it up and went to see a different kind of doctor – a chiropractor. During our consultation, she declared that no one should have scoliosis and that she could get my spine straight. Why I didn't do a heel turn and walk out of her office immediately is beyond me. My spine will always have a scoliosis, it may decrease in curvature, but it will always be present. If someone promises you a straight spine, you need to politely bid your adieu.

The consult was at 4 p.m. in the afternoon and I'd been with my two, wildly energetic boys, ages two and four, all day long. The chiropractor said she needed to do some X-rays and study them before we started treatment. I'm pretty sure I'd expended all my usable brain cells for the day and obliged to her request. I wasn't given a gown and she told me I didn't need to take my bra or belt off. I agreed and went with her. I honestly think I was too worried about my kids running into the X-ray area to realize I was *again* taking X-rays without wearing a sports bra and workout pants. So, *again* I got X-rays with metal in them.

My jaw hit the check out desk when I was given a $350 bill for the initial visit and X-rays. I was not told that my insurance wouldn't cover X-rays at a chiropractic office and only covered a portion of the consult visit. I was too far down the rabbit's hole to stop now. I booked my next appointment.

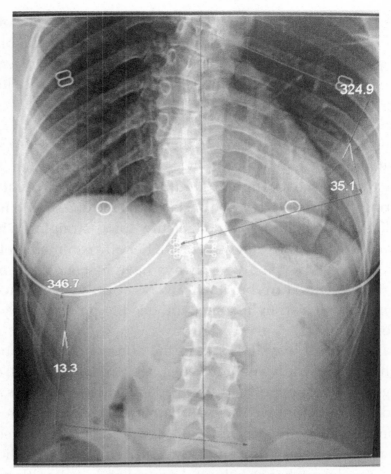

This chiropractor's X-ray of my back was taken from the front, so it looks like I have an upper left curve instead of an upper right. You can see the Cobb Angle measurements added in.

The chiropractor was nervous to tell me what my curvature degrees were since it'd been a year since my last X-ray with the orthopedist and she thought the degree was pretty bad. My upper curve was at 35 degrees and my lower curve was at 13 degrees. I was elated, much to the chiropractor's surprise. Yes, my upper curve had increased by four degrees but my lower curve decreased by 10 degrees. *Awesome!* Now remember, I'd been hauling my two little boys around for the entire day by the time I had those X-rays. If I had done my exercises, had a massage the night before, had early morning X-rays, and hadn't been carrying my kids around, who knows how low my curvature degrees would be! Truly, I bet my upper curve is still around 31 degrees, if not a degree or two lower. Heavens only knows about my lower curve. Could it really be living in the single digits?!

The chiropractor snapped her adjusting tool up and down my spine, but I didn't allow her to manually crack my neck. I drew the line on that one. She had me lay down in a few certain positions with pillows under me for a few minutes (mind you, I'd been doing this on my own already) and then I was off. I saw her maybe a few more times until I pulled the plug. My emotions were all over the board during the week of doing her treatments. The constant adjusting of my spine was really messing with my nervous system. I was in a lot of back pain by her adjustments, and quite frankly, I knew it wasn't good for my body.

Interestingly, I saw one of my regular masseuses shortly after my last chiropractic treatment, and she noted that my muscular and fascial system hadn't been that bad in years. Lesson learned. Another doctor bites the dust.

As I've said many times in this book, every scoliotic back is different. For this reason, particularly while you are going through puberty or other bodily changes, I would highly suggest you find an orthopedist you trust in your area to walk alongside you. If a curve worsens by five degrees in a period of three to six months, the orthopedist is going to carefully watch it to make sure it doesn't continue on that roller coaster path. That five degree increase could change the orthopedist's choice of treatment to ensure the spine doesn't continue to spiral into itself.

With scoliosis, the main reason medical intervention takes place is to make sure organs don't become compromised. The lungs and heart can be squished by the rotation of the rib cage. The rib bones can start to push into these vital organs and decrease their ability to function.

Another reason medical intervention can take place is to address neurological issues. Decrease in leg or arm function and nerve pain can be red flags that neurological issues may be at hand. The nervous system is not something to be toyed with, so orthopedic intervention needs to happen.

I received a phone call from a physical therapist in town befuddled and frustrated by a seven-year-old female patient's scoliosis. She'd worked with her for a few months but had not seen any positive results. She had an upper left curve of 42 degrees. Four red flags hit me right off the bat:

1. She's quite young to be diagnosed with scoliosis.

2. If she's small-framed, she's more than likely not hitting puberty early, (which can initiate spinal changes due to hormones).

3. The degree of her curve is very high, especially for being so young.

4. Her scoliosis curved to the left, not to the right, which is the norm.

She was complaining of left chest pain to the physical therapist. I told the physical therapist that spiral spines usually curve away from the heart, leaving the heart space to function properly. In this case, her scoliosis was curving into her heart.

Red flag. I don't know if that was the cause of her chest pain, but I do know it's certainly not going to help.

The physical therapist received permission from the patient's mother to consult with me about her daughter and show me CT images taken of her daughter's spine. Immediately I notice that this little girl had a hemi-vertebrae. She had congenital scoliosis – exercise won't help, only surgery. After studying it a little more, I notice that she had roughly four vertebrae that were fused together from her bony structure in the deep curve. Questions start piling up in my head.

A surgeon doesn't usually order a CT scan unless he sees an issue in an X-ray. Why did he allow the mom to "try physical therapy" if he knew it wasn't going to work? Why did the physical therapist not look at the CT scan until after working with the girl for months proving no progress? Why did I, who am not a doctor, see the genetic anomalies in this little girl's spine and not someone with a doctorate degree? Most likely, these spinal issues happened in utero, so why didn't the ultrasound technicians catch it when the mom was pregnant? Why didn't her pediatrician catch it *before* the age of seven, because it must have been there from birth? Why didn't her parent's catch it earlier?

I noticed on one of the CT scans that her two top ribs were really close together and asked the physical therapist if she'd complained of nerve pain in her right hand. The physical therapist said that yes, she had been having issues with moving her thumb properly, and had recently seen an orthopedist. The doctor said she was most likely missing a muscle in her thumb and offered to do surgery on it. The physical therapist put two-and-two together and excitedly proclaimed, "It's because of the scoliosis! Her two top ribs are pinching nerves causing her right thumb to not work!" Naturally, I agreed with her diagnosis.

Why is a large part of our medical world living in the dark ages in regards to scoliosis? What are medical schools teaching people? So much wasted time. So much wasted money - most producing no positive results. Does all this not seem like medical malpractice to anyone else? With an estimated five to seven million people living with scoliosis in America, one would think that the medical community would have a better grasp on it.

No matter what form of scoliosis you have, the reality is that there is no cure for it. Surgery doesn't even fix scoliosis. You exchange one abnormality for another – a mobile curved spine for a non-mobile (almost) straight spine. After surgery, there is usually some curve left, the rotation won't have been fully fixed, and the spine is fused so it can't move. The moral of the story is, if medical intervention is absolutely necessary, take the appropriate action to live a long and happy life. For the rest of us, we must make peace with our scoliosis and learn how to own it.

Most people's scoliosis is never severe enough for a back brace or surgery (and thank God for that!). So what do you do if you have more than a 10-degree curve but less than 40?

The usual treatment for scoliosis in the medical world is as follows:

- 10-25 degree curve: observation
- 25-40 degree curve: brace
- 40+ degree curve: surgery

Know that there are always exceptions. For example, a brace is usually only given to an adolescent who hasn't finished growing. So, for an adult with scoliosis, the observation period would extend to about 40 degrees. Sometimes surgery isn't suggested until a curve is greater than 50, so an adult might remain in the observation period until their curve is at least 50 degrees.

With the possible exception of physical therapy (that is, IF your physician will write you a prescription/referral, IF your insurance will cover the therapy, and IF you can find a physical therapist who specializes in scoliosis), there's little for the medical world to do for you, unless you are an adolescent and your back is deemed bad enough for a brace. So, the medical community just watches and waits...they observe. My goal is for your scoliosis to never progress to the point where you need to consider a brace or surgery.

The reality is physicians are very limited in their treatment options for scoliosis. There are less severe and less drastic treatments for scoliosis than bracing and surgery, but you need to look outside of the medical world for those – and you must know specifically what to look for.

6) be proactive

For the record, "observation" is not a treatment. While your orthopedist is treating you by "observation," you must be proactive in areas outside of the orthopedic world.

Over the years, I have patiently and empathetically listened as parents tell a nearly identical story over and over again, and it goes something like this:

> "My daughter went in for her yearly check-up and the doctor said she has scoliosis. My stomach immediately tied up into knots and I anxiously asked the doctor what I could do to fix it. He said, 'I'd like to get X-rays of her back. It doesn't look bad enough for surgery or bracing yet, so we'll most likely just observe it over the next few years.'"

My response? Be proactive! It is a HUGE blessing that you are simply in the observation period. Do something about it so you never progress past that point. A surgeon went to school to learn how to perform surgery. So, if you go to an orthopedic surgeon he will most likely tell you if and when he can perform surgery. He is most likely *not* going to suggest you go to a

Pilates lesson with him two times a week to see if that will decrease your curvature and decrease the pain. Surgery is where his expertise lies. If your orthopedist suggests you try body practitioners, or even refers you to a few good ones, stay with that orthopedist!

What do I mean by being proactive about scoliosis? Now is the time to try out different kinds of movement therapies by different kinds of body practitioners in your area. One thing I learned early on when working with scoliosis clients is that every body is *extremely* different. You have to find a practitioner who understands *your* body.

Here are some suggestions as to forms of therapy you can explore to help manage your scoliosis. Each form is described briefly, as some of these therapies may be unfamiliar to you:

- GYROTONIC® Method: A form of exercise which is characterized by circular and spiraling movements that help with three-dimensional awareness and increase functional capacity of the spine. Exercises are performed on the GYROTONIC® Pulley Tower.

- Myofascial therapy: This form of massage is specifically aimed at releasing dysfunctional soft tissue, or fascia, in the body. Myofascial Release, Rolfing, and Structural Integration are three ways you may hear myofascial therapy described.

- Pilates: A form of exercise that focuses on correct spinal and pelvic alignment to develop a strong core and increase overall flexibility. Many different specialized pieces of equipment are used, such as the Reformer, Cadillac, Chair, and Barrel.

- Schroth Method physical therapy: A form of scoliosis-specific physical therapy designed to decrease spinal curvature and rotation. Inpatient and outpatient clinics are scattered around the world. The main Schroth clinic is in Germany.

Truly, there are so many other kinds of therapy that could help. I've heard of people having success with yoga, acupuncture, neuromuscular and trigger point massage, and even neurologists who specialize in scoliosis. If you find an extremely skilled therapist, under a broad array of different therapies, they quite possibly could positively affect your scoliosis. The most important point I want to get across is that you need to find someone *in your town* who can work with you.

I was asked in an interview who my scoliosis "dream team" of fitness and medical professionals would consist of. It was a really loaded question because I truly believe that the most important part of successful scoliosis movement therapy is *being seen weekly* by a good movement practitioner, who really understands scoliosis. While there can be wonderful benefits to flying to an intensive, multi-week scoliosis therapy clinic every year, I can't stress enough the importance of also having an in-town practitioner who knows your body.

All that your spiral spine needs is a few weeks of the perfect storm to twist your spine up tightly. If you are a tween or teenaged girl, that perfect storm could be a growth spurt, hormone changes, very little bodily movement from sitting in a desk all day, carrying a 20-pound backpack on your back, etc. If you are an adult, it could be sleepless nights from dealing with a newborn or ill child or grandchild, dealing with a bodily illness of your own, the weather being less than ideal outside so you're stuck inside with not much bodily movement, an emotionally traumatic experience happening in the family, hormonal changes, etc. You need someone who can catch the perfect storm in its tracks, while it's happening, and stop the havoc it's wreaking.

I'll expand on the scoliosis dream team question by elaborating a bit more on my personal story. As you know, I live in the Nashville, TN area. I love it and so do a lot of others. You never know what famous person will be sitting next to you at a coffee shop, dropping off their kid at school next to you in carline, or popping into your Pilates studio. We've got a Tiffany's, Louis Vuitton, Nordstrom's, and Whole Foods, just to name a few of the high-end amenities in town.

On top of Nashville being known as Music City, it's also one of the largest healthcare towns in the world. One would think with the combination of affluence and being a healthcare worldly hub that there would be some great medical people to tend to those living with scoliosis. Think again.

I've yet to find an orthopedist I like who can track my spiral spine. I'd love to work with a Schroth physical therapist, but there aren't any in Nashville. The closest one is a three-hour drive away. I've contacted him multiple times, but have never received a reply via email or phone. I even called the clinic where he works, explained my situation, and asked if I could book up all his morning appointments because I'd be traveling from three hours away. The receptionist explained that he only schedules 30-minute appointments. Another door closed in my face.

Even with all my training, I'll never be able to go through Schroth training because I'm not a physical therapist. My husband and I have even contemplated me going to PT school to get my doctorate so I could be Schroth-trained. Once we reviewed all the pros and cons, we actually laughed out loud because it simply didn't make any sense. I make a good living, have a full client load, and am very happy in my current teaching conditions. It just didn't make sense to spend tens of thousands of dollars on a doctorate degree to pretty much do what I'm already doing.

I'm a body practitioner, and most of my current clientele has scoliosis. Note that I did not go looking for scoliosis clients, they sought me out. Luckily, I've researched, read, studied, practiced, and watched the heck out of every piece of scoliosis material I could get my hands on. I think I take very good care of my clients.

What about people all over the world living in towns smaller than Nashville? What kind of practitioners are living in those small towns? Maybe a basic personal trainer and perhaps a massage therapist might live within a 50-mile radius of the town. You might find a physical therapist at a medical facility nearby, but more than likely, they won't be Schroth-trained. Are there people living with scoliosis in small town? Absolutely. How are they supposed to better manage their scoliosis?

Let's go to a little bit bigger town, but not yet as big as Nashville. I bet there are Pilates instructors, maybe even some who've worked with scoliosis clients before. Actually, I get emails from instructors all over the world telling me that a large part of their clientele has scoliosis. So many people have turned to body practitioners to help them with their scoliosis.

So, back to the scoliosis dream team question. I don't want to create a fictitious, unattainable scenario for anyone living with scoliosis. My best suggestion is to do your research and find the highest educated practitioner you can get your hands on *in your own town*. If need be, help them get additional training on how to work on your spiral spine. Help them help your scoliosis.

If you are working with a body practitioner who needs a bit more training on how to work with your spiral spine, there are some good continuing education courses they can attend. I've also created many teaching products for body practitioners available on SpiralSpine.com.

If you live in a town where multiple practitioners are available, you may choose to use a multitude of them to help your back like I, and many of my clients do. No matter what type of practitioner you choose, the key to successful scoliosis therapy is finding an experienced body practitioner who has in-depth anatomical knowledge and a good grasp on scoliosis.

Scoliosis affects the entire body through different systems such as the bony system, the muscular system, and the fascial system. Using very elementary descriptions, I'll attempt to briefly describe how these systems are affected by scoliosis.

The bony system is the frame on which the muscular and fascial systems live. When you see an X-ray of a spiral spine, you are looking at bone. In some scoliosis cases, the actual bones of the spine have not changed shape, but are simply unevenly stacked on top of one another. In other cases, one or multiple vertebra don't fit the picture of what a usual bone in the spine looks like. If a vertebra is a different shape, other bones up and down the body will be affected. The bony system is usually what orthopedists attempt to affect with bracing or surgery.

The muscular system is what makes our bodies move. Muscles have the ability to contract, release, and stretch. The scoliotic spine affects the muscular system because the distance between certain bones changes due to the sideways curving and rotation. Certain muscles must then change their length due to that bony change.

Muscles pull on bones, they don't push. So, if certain muscles are in an area of the back where the bones are closer together due to the scoliosis curve, the muscles are going to stay in a short, bound position. They don't have much of an opportunity to stretch. On the opposite side of the spine, those same muscles live in a constant stretched or long position and it's going to be harder for them to contract because of their length. The bone/muscle relationship is a bit of a catch-22 because unless intervention takes place, the short muscles keep getting shorter and more bound, which causes the scoliotic bones to stay where they are or even twist up more. It's a vicious cycle. The muscular system is one of the systems that body practitioners can attempt to functionally improve.

The fascial system hasn't been given nearly enough attention in the scoliotic community, in my opinion. It hasn't been until the last decade or so that hard, medical research has shown how important fascia is to correcting bodily ailments. Fascia is a fancy word for connective tissue. There are many, many different forms of fascia throughout the body. Fascia encases and intertwines muscles, organs, joint systems...it wraps the entire body.

When certain parts of your fascia receive the brunt of trauma (and you better believe that your fascial system has received trauma from your spiral spine), the entire bodily fascial system is affected. Remember my story about the older gentlemen, Ted? Remember how he had a number of ailments and surgeries all over his body except for his scoliotic spine? I would put money down that he never did therapy on his traumatized scoliotic fascial system. That, in turn, could have been a partial cause for the rest of his bodily pains, injuries, and surgeries. Fascia is another bodily system that body practitioners can attempt to functionally improve.

When taking the exercise path for therapy, you need to expect results from your practitioners. Together, set clear, reasonable goals to see if your exercise or massage regimen is working. Most therapeutic regimens are not covered by insurance. If you are with a skilled practitioner, you will most likely be paying $50-$100 an hour for a private session. This therapeutic approach not only takes money, but it also takes time and dedication to stay on a disciplined schedule. If goals are not being achieved and your scoliosis is worsening, then you may need to seek medical attention. Do not continue to needlessly spend valuable time and money if your plan of action is not working.

On the other hand, don't give up too soon. Be patient. You'll most likely be taking baby steps. On multiple occasions, I've had people come to see me for a private lesson (and even drop-in on a group class of mine) and leave after the first lesson frustrated because their scoliosis wasn't "fixed." I don't think they understood the all-encompassing scope of scoliosis. You must do your research and from there, set reasonable goals. If a non-medical, therapeutic approach does work for you, as it has for many people all over the world, you may reduce the likelihood that you will ever need a brace or have surgery. How awesome would that be?!?

I must say a cautionary word when sifting through exercise instructors and therapists. I have seen a trend going on with fitness professionals who do not understand scoliosis, let alone know how to correctly work with scoliosis clients. On more than one occasion, I've told an instructor before a class I was taking that I have scoliosis and their response was simply, "That's OK, everyone has scoliosis. Just keep up the best you can and take a break when you need to." If you ever receive a response like this, please do not continue working with that person. Keep doing your research and find a better-educated body practitioner.

Here are potential goals to set with your body practitioner(s):

- In six months, at my next scoliosis X-ray appointment, my curve will have decreased.
  - You may choose a reasonable decrease in degree or just be content that it has decreased, even if only slightly.
- Within the next six months, my scoliosis pain will have decreased.
  - I do need to add that muscle discomfort from exercise is not scoliosis pain. If you have never exercised before, then you will need to learn to differentiate "scoliosis pain" from "working out pain."
- My body practitioner will measure my scoliosis with a scoliometer every lesson to make sure my scoliotic rotation is not increasing.
  - Getting a reading from a scoliometer is not as exact as getting a measurement by a medical professional from an X-ray. However, on twisted days, a scoliometer is a nice tool to keep on-hand to make sure your scoliosis isn't winding up too much. I measure my scoliosis clients at the beginning and end of every session to see how their body responded to the stretches and exercises I had them do.
- Within four months, I will be able to see a visual, physical change in musculature in my back to better support my spine.
- Within six months, my posture will have significantly improved.

- This, in turn, could increase self-image. Depending on your specific scoliosis, the degree in curvature may not decrease but your entire body doesn't have to emit the look of pain and self-woe.

The tough reality is that no one knows for sure if your curve will stay the same for the rest of your life or if it will progress. Educated guesses can be made, but no one really knows for sure. Corrective movement therapy, in its many forms, is one of the only approach that can possibly decrease a curve without spinal fusion surgery. If you find that corrective movement therapy isn't helping your curve, then you can simply change your mind and stop. Your entire body will be stronger and you'll have gained more knowledge about your body along the way. Just keep gathering information to find the best techniques that help your spiral spine stay mobile.

Be willing to experiment on yourself. All of the options I mentioned are good for your health, regardless if you have scoliosis. Find the routine that works for you. That regimen may need to change next year as your body changes. Be willing to stay flexible (no pun intended). Commit to keeping your body healthy. Be proactive about your spiral spine health. Take action.

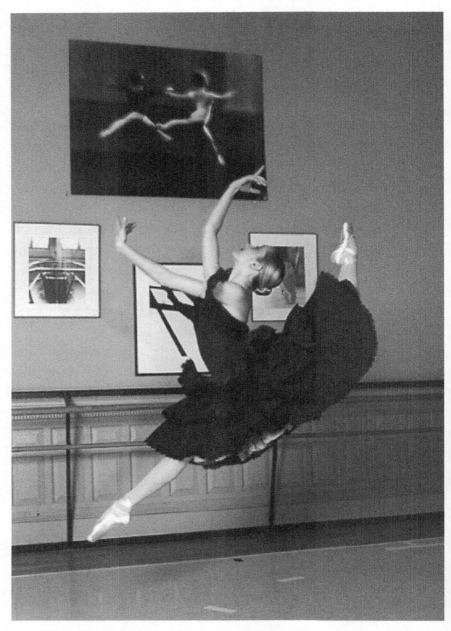

This was taken of me in high school in 1991. No wonder my mom doubted the doctor's initial scoliosis diagnosis! She figured there was no way someone with a spiral spine could dance like I did.

7

a mother's story

This chapter has been specially-written by my mother, SuzAnne Weston-Kirkegaard. Who better to encourage a parent whose child has been diagnosed with scoliosis than a mother whose daughter was diagnosed with it?

Somewhere near the end of her middle school years, Erin was diagnosed with scoliosis. It's significant that I can't remember this date because I'm usually really good with dates, especially when it comes to my children. You see, I'm a "mama bear." I put my kids in every activity I could find for them to try. We went on many family vacations, they tried all types of food, and I took them every year for their routine check-ups.

During one of these routine check-ups, our pediatrician asked me if I thought Erin might have scoliosis. My immediate answer was an emphatic, "There's NO way!" My daughter was a very serious and dedicated dancer! She had danced for at least 10 years by that time and was in a disciplined ballet program. No way could she do any of that extreme dance stuff and have scoliosis.

Our pediatrician was the only pediatrician the kids had ever seen and I trusted him completely, but when he brought up the scoliosis question I was sure he had lost his mind. So he let the issue drop, possibly because I seemed so alarmed.

Another year passed and when it came time for physicals again, the pediatrician brought it up a little more forcefully and asked me to look at Erin from the back when she bent over to touch her toes. You could see how her back was higher on one side and slightly curved. He then asked her to stand upright and square off her shoulders. The result was one shoulder blade was pulled out towards me! I even wondered if she could be forcing that goofy position. When did that happen and how come I hadn't noticed it before? I felt like a horrible mom. How could I have missed this!?

The next thing I remember was the pediatrician asking Erin if her back hurt and she said that sometimes it did, if she danced a lot. Had I ignored the pain in her back? The doctor kept assuring me, "We're just gathering information." We left that appointment with a referral slip to a spinal specialist and another slip for a set of X-rays.

"Information gathering" is what I had to hang my hat on. I was scared. I was scared for my daughter. Would she have to get a brace? Would she have to have back surgery? I blew off what the pediatrician said last year about her back. If I had caught it last year would it have been this bad now? How did her twisted spine sneak up on me? The questions and self-doubt started piling up in my head.

Thinking back on that initial diagnosis, I was convinced the specialist would laugh at the crazy notion that my daughter had scoliosis. First of all, I had done everything I could think of to keep her healthy and active. Second of all, people who had an ailment (like those with scoliosis) simply couldn't do the things Erin could do or dance the way she could dance. Or so I thought.

The specialist took a good look at her X-rays and said, "Yep, she's got scoliosis. She's got an 'S' curve and it's measuring at 17 degrees. If it hurts her enough or she gets to 20 degrees, we'll talk about her wearing a brace or surgery." I couldn't believe what he was saying! He went on to say that he wasn't sure but there might be some hairline fractures in some of the vertebrae and he wasn't sure about the source of those. "Maybe dance or maybe scoliosis," he said. She was supposed to rest for a week and, if the pain was gone, she could dance again. He also stated that she was very lucky she was a serious dancer because it had kept her strong and flexible. We never saw that specialist again.

I felt like my head was spinning with a million questions all pointing to this being my fault! I didn't know what to do. Usually, I was very self-assured and confident when it came to decisions about my children.

The pediatrician continued to watch her spine and once even said she would probably be a whole inch taller if her spine wasn't curved. That comment made me feel like I must be the worst mother in the world. But, none of that information or my anxiety seemed to stop Erin and I'm so grateful for that. She continued to reach for her goals like nothing could stop her.

It was during the years she danced with the Rockettes that it truly hit home for me that she had scoliosis. She had a lot of knee pain, foot pain, back pain, and shoulder pain. How could anyone with a damaged spine dance like she did? What had I done to encourage her to pursue this dance dream? Should I have kept her from dancing? Had I been hiding my head in the sand? Should she have had the surgery or worn a brace? The questions kept spinning, but I couldn't turn back time. I made the best decision I could with the information I had.

Erin had been diagnosed with scoliosis and I felt terribly guilty. We didn't know how or when she got it. Eventually, what we did realize was that Erin was pursuing her passion and dreams even though her spine wasn't perfectly straight. Encourage your child to do the same. I learned from Erin that scoliosis doesn't have to be a handicap. Even though it wasn't my fault she had scoliosis, I felt responsible and helpless. My beautiful daughter would face spinal challenges for her entire life and I felt like it was my fault.

As with many things in life, time and communication seem to heal and make things better. Watching and talking with my daughter as she made her journey through this challenge has brought me to the realization that I should not be playing the blame game with myself. Just as Erin had to learn to own her scoliosis, I had to learn to not own her scoliosis. I had to learn to overcome my guilt.

Now I know that it's not the challenges we face that make us who we are, it's the way we deal with those challenges. Scoliosis was just an inconvenience for Erin. One passion led to the next and now she trains people who face the same obstacle she does. It's not about having scoliosis, it's about how you deal with it. You get to decide what you will do with scoliosis. I am so proud of what Erin has accomplished with Spiral Spine.

8) a final thought

When I was a dancer, my scoliosis was an inconvenience. As my back discomfort increased, I had to learn to manage my pain, which gave me a challenge. How on earth was I going to cope with the bodily ramifications that scoliosis was giving me? When I came into my own as a Pilates instructor, I realized my scoliosis was a gift that had been given to me so I could help others understand and work through their own spiral spines. It's so interesting how an inconvenience, which morphed into a challenge, and ended as a gift, could wind up simply being a small piece of a bigger journey.

Now, I'm a mom. It's my turn to collect all the information and make the best decisions for my children as they face life's challenges. My sons don't have scoliosis (yet), so I thankfully haven't had to walk alongside them on that challenging path, but I've had my share of issues with my youngest son, Asher.

During the year when Asher was between ages one and two, his body went haywire and no one in the medical world could figure out what was happening. I brought Asher from one specialist to the next. He was diagnosed with an anaphylactic peanut allergy, had a lot of hearing and speech issues, constantly had dermatological problems, and had multiple ear infections treated with round after round of oral antibiotics. He ended up in surgery to get tubes put in his ears, and two weeks later ended up with a staph infection. I drug my feet with each diagnosis, desiring some sort of a connection between everything and the root cause of it all.

After a year of expensive treatments, multiple doctors, a surgery for Asher, mounds of prescribed medication, and no hard root causes to show for all this chaos, I was thoroughly finished with the path we were on. I pulled him from every single doctor he was seeing.

Our new pediatrician did food sensitivity testing and found Asher had many sensitivities. We pulled all those particular foods from his diet and went to an organic paleo diet. We learned to buy and cook in new ways. Our whole family had to learn to eat differently. When he'd get an ear infection, we would use remedies that wouldn't harm his already leaky intestines. I started researching intestinal issues like it was my job and acting on what I learned. We started a large organic garden in our backyard so we had more fresh produce readily available. I listened to hundreds of hours of online lectures by doctors and functional medicine practitioners all over the world. It was an overwhelming task I assigned to myself, but the train was gradually beginning to move in the right direction for Asher. I was determined to increase the quality of my son's health, and as a blessed and unexpected gift, the health of the rest of the family was improving as well.

While I was slowly but surely putting all the pieces together for Asher's body, I wasn't tending to my own emotional health. The emotional baggage I carried wasn't going away. My mother's guilt was incessant. I was his caretaker, his mother. I felt like I had foolishly listened to doctors' advice without getting second and third opinions and my little son received the brunt of those decisions. Thoughts like, "if I just realized what was happening earlier," or "if I had just done my research before giving him all those antibiotics," kept circulating in my mind. The "if I would have, then…" thoughts kept coming. Asher had a much more difficult first few years of life than his older brother and I absolutely felt like I was the one to blame. Both of my boys came from my body, so I thought I must be at fault for one having a more arduous journey than the other.

On a particularly dark emotional day for me battling with Asher's health, it occurred to me that the scope of emotions a parent of a child with scoliosis goes through is massive. Asher will most likely have no long-term ramifications from his first few years of life, but those diagnosed with scoliosis have it forever. I have so much empathy to offer families coping with the life-long journey of scoliosis. It's emotionally draining and you have to be committed for the long haul. Just like I had to make peace with my scoliosis, I had to make peace with Asher's myriad of health issues. I had to lay my heartache and guilt over Asher's problems at the feet of my Heavenly Father. It's an on-going conversation I still have with God. My burden is lightening as I continually learn to release it, and I am so thankful for that.

Asher is older now, has no anaphylactic peanut allergy and his speech has improved immensely. He recently had another surgery, but I'd done extensive research after the last one and was at peace with the path he was now on. When most people meet Asher, they just see an energetic, hilarious, and sweet boy. That makes my heart so happy. They don't see my "parental mistakes." They don't see his past health struggles. They see a younger brother that can give his older brother, by all of 21 months, a run for his money. They see one half of a dynamic duo that family and friends call the Myers Family Circus.

As you can see, my life has not been very quiet over the last few years. I had so many issues to assess and deal with for my family, and yet I still had my spiral spine to manage. I'll always have my scoliosis to manage, which is why my husband and I made some important life changes so I can better own my scoliosis. We've reprioritized energy, time, and money to help my body function at its optimal potential.

A few years ago we moved houses, and I now have a private studio in our home where I have Pilates and GYROTONIC® equipment. If I wake up at 5:30 a.m., after being up with a sick kid in the middle of the night and my body is hurting, I can grab a cup of tea and get on my equipment to align myself. When my kids are napping, I can go into the studio to make my body supple and strong. I realized a while ago that with little kids, I was going to have next to zero personal time, so my husband and I made some huge life changes. My entire family has a better quality of life because of the changes we made. Now, my kids ask if they can exercise with me. What an awesome consequence of changing our priorities around!

I have myofascial therapy about every three weeks and a trigger point massage every few months. My schedule is so crazy, that sometimes I'll go to the masseuse's studio, sometimes her house, or sometimes she'll come to my house depending on what else is happening with other family members. No one cares about my spinal health more than me, so I just have to make time for it…even if that means kids are playing under the massage table.

I had to figure out a way to get my heart rate up because I realized my spiral spine doesn't like it when I run. My scoliosis doesn't like the compression and my ribcage and spinal musculature gets too bound after running. So, I've found that I love to rollerblade, which I can do in my neighborhood. If I can get to the gym, I like to work on the elliptical and ride on a stationary bike. Every few weeks I'll drop into a yoga class. I constantly switch studios, teachers, and styles of yoga to challenge my body in new ways.

Every few years, I get a new movement certification to keep challenging my body to move in new ways. My mind is also challenged this way because I'm forced to look at the human body from another perspective.

Since my plate has become so extremely full, I've had to learn to switch my focus to that of a laser beam in regards to my health. While a fluorescent light bulb can light a room, a laser beam that takes the same amount of energy but is just focused on one particular spot, can cut through metal. My exercise, food, and spiritual life are all extremely intentional. I make sure my physical activities make me strong and flexible, which will help and not damage my scoliosis. The food I put in my body heals me and doesn't harm me. I'm acutely aware of where my mind is. I focus on the One who is the Light of the world, so I do not walk in darkness.

My scoliosis hasn't made my life bad. Actually, I'd say I'm pretty darn blessed. My scoliosis has led me to a much more intentional life. I don't know what lies ahead for my back, but I do know that I will continue to do everything in my power to keep my scoliosis from progressing. As for my children, I hope they don't end up with scoliosis. But, if they do, I'll be there to help their physical bodies as I pray for emotional strength. Regardless of what happens, I will always think backs are beautiful, just like I did all those years ago as a teenager in ballet class.

I love and appreciate my spiral spine, and I hope that one day, you will come to love and appreciate yours, too.

about the author
Erin Myers

Erin Myers is a Pilates and fitness professional who has dedicated her career to the creation of Spiral Spine, a series of resources designed to inform, inspire, and ignite the scoliosis community. Diagnosed with scoliosis as a teenager, she was told by her physician to 'watch and wait,' while she continued dancing at an elite level. When she was 21 years old, Erin went on tour with the Radio City Rockettes but soon began suffering debilitating knee and back pain.

Thankfully, her world changed forever when an instructor challenged her to try Pilates. She quickly noticed that the muscles around her knees began to strengthen in ways that had never been possible before, and her back responded just as favorably. In fact, she was pain-free! Intrigued, Erin began researching the affects of movement on the scoliotic back.

Research proved surprisingly hard to come by, but over time, Erin gathered a substantial amount of information and began to see firsthand how individual bodies responded to specialized movement and massage. And the physical and emotional relief that movement provided was undeniable. She was driven to begin spreading the word, by embracing her own *beautiful scoliotic back*.

Moving from NYC to Nashville, Erin established a successful Pilates studio and became known for her personalized work with scoliosis clients. After a mere four years of ownership, she sold her Pilates studio for six-times its earnings, and now consults and teaches on a private basis, in addition to overseeing Spiral Spine.

Trained in Pilates at the Kane School of Core Integration in NYC, Erin is certified in the GYROTONIC® Method, holds certifications by the American Council on Exercise and the Pilates Method Alliance, and is a teaching faculty member of Balanced Body. She holds a Bachelor's degree in Managerial Entrepreneurship from Pace University in NYC (Cum Laude).

Erin also works periodically with Centric Health Resources creating fitness programs for extremely rare genetic diseases for their patient wellness program. She continues to teach Pilates teacher training and Pilates continuing education.

Erin lives in Brentwood, TN, with her husband, Aaron, and their two sons, Levi and Asher. Her goal is simply to inspire others affected by scoliosis by sharing her own journey, and encouraging them to take charge of their own physical and emotional health.

The Myers Family, 2014.

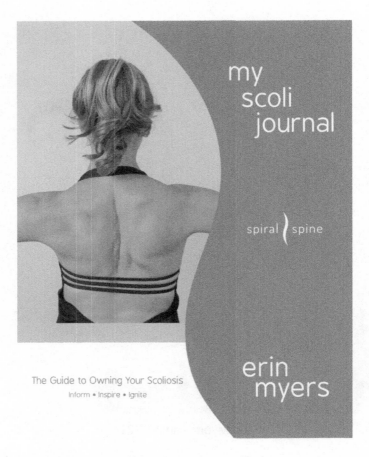

The Guide to Owning Your Scoliosis
Inform • Inspire • Ignite

my scoli journal

spiral spine

erin myers

Scoliosis can be a source of physical and emotional anguish for everyone it touches. *My Scoli Journal* will help you express your thoughts and feelings in a meaningful and positive way, guiding you towards a full, pain-free life.

There's no need to let your scoliosis own you. Learn how to own it! *My Scoli Journal* will show you how.

Available from Amazon.com and other retail outlets

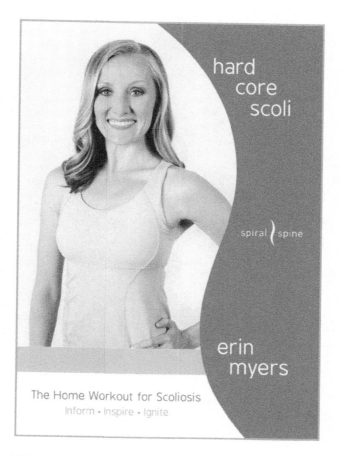

hard core scoli

spiral) spine

erin myers

The Home Workout for Scoliosis
Inform • Inspire • Ignite

Did you know it's possible to get a great workout while improving your scoliosis? This 40 minute workout brings Erin Myers' deep knowledge of both scoliosis and core strengthening straight to your living room. Basic items found around the house are used to increase awareness of body alignment, making this workout accessible to everyone.

Take control of your quality of life and strengthen your Spiral Spine with *Hard Core Scoli*.

Available from Amazon.com and other retail outlets

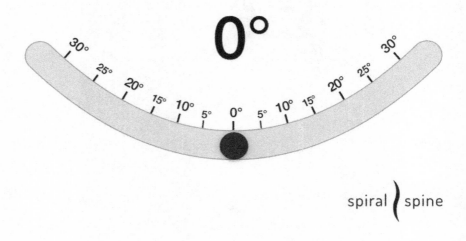

The Scoliometer by Spiral Spine is a simple, easy-to-use app that gives users the ability to measure their ribcage and vertebral rotation from the comfort of their own home. With regular use of the scoliometer, users can determine which therapies help decrease their spinal rotation.

The Scoliometer by Spiral Spine can be
purchased online at itunes.apple.com

Made in the USA
Las Vegas, NV
04 January 2024

83931686R00059